Alkaline Foods: An Alkaline Cookbook For Balancing Your pH And Improving Your Health Quickly And Easily

Disclaimer and Terms of Use: Effort has been made to ensure that the information in this book is accurate and complete, however, the author and the publisher do not warrant the accuracy of the information, text and graphics contained within the book due to the rapidly changing nature of science, research, known and unknown facts and internet. The Author and the publisher do not hold any responsibility for errors, omissions or contrary interpretation of the subject matter herein. This book is presented solely for motivational and informational purposes only.

Table of Contents

Introduction

The internal environment of our body is alkaline with a pH slightly above 7.0. Our body organs will be able to work more efficiently at this pH. The immunological and repair mechanisms of our body will be at its best at this pH. However, the metabolic reactions and biochemical process occurring in our body produces different types of acids. We produce acids in our body when we exercise, when we breathe and when we digest the food we eat. The various chemical reactions occurring in our body occur within the specific pH of 7.0. Hence our body tries to maintain the normal pH level by eliminating the acidic products formed by different metabolic processes. Our body needs alkaline mineral salts to buffer or neutralize the acids formed in our body. So, it is necessary to have an alkaline diet, if you want to improve the health.

Our body has the blood pH between 7.35 and 7.45. By eating alkaline foods, we help our body to maintain this pH level. This does not mean that one has to avoid acidic foods completely. We have to keep a balance of acidic and alkaline food so that our body will be able to maintain the pH balance with less effort. The diet most of us have contains processed sugars, refined grains, artificial sweeteners, etc. causes the formation of acids in our body. When these foods are combined with psychological stress, lack of exercise, lack of sleep results in various degenerative diseases.

Why Is It Necessary To Have Alkaline Foods?

All foods have alkaline and acid forming elements in them. It is not the organic part of the food that determines its acidity or alkalinity but the inorganic part like the calcium, sodium, potassium, magnesium, sulfur and phosphorus determines whether it forms acidic or alkaline residues once they get burned by the metabolic processes. Eating too much of acid-forming foods can affect your health badly. When the body is unable to get the nutrients for maintaining the pH from the food we eat, body tend to absorb it from the vital tissues and bones. This will reduce the ability of the body to repair and detoxify itself. This will make the body more vulnerable to different illnesses and fatigue. It has been found that the alkaline diet improves digestion, prevents mood swings and improves the skin appearance. Metabolic acidity has adverse effect on the cell metabolism causing impaired production of energy, fluid accumulation in the body, increased production of free radicals. Acidic condition in the internal environment of the body leads to loss of bone minerals, reduction in the production of growth hormones, loss of muscle mass and development of stones in kidneys.

The Benefits Of Having An Alkaline Diet

- Alkaline diet improves digestion and reduces flatulence and bloating of the abdomen

- Alkaline diet contains seeds and nuts and vegetables and fruits which help to improve the skin tone. The essential fatty acids in these food items keep the skin nourished.

- This diet controls the blood sugar levels of the body and this result in increased ability to focus and concentrate and to have better memory.

- The grains included in this diet contain serotonin in high levels and this will help the person to remain happy as the serotonin receptor sites get satisfied.

- Having an alkaline diet will help to prevent infections. Bacteria, fungi and yeast that cause infections in our body thrive well in an acidic environment. Acidic environment reduces the number of good bacteria in your body and you will be prone to develop infections.

- The energy level of the person gets greatly improved as these alkaline foods release the carbohydrates slowly into the system which keeps the blood sugar level balanced.

- As this diet contains fruits and vegetables containing fibers, it makes you feel full and there will not be cravings for food or sugar.

- This diet will help to maintain a healthy weight. As the diet contains fruits, vegetables and whole grains the cravings are less and hence there are less chances for over eating. Moreover these foods do not contain excess sugar or carbohydrates which will cause weight gain.

- Alkaline diet will reduce the risk of developing cancer. When our body becomes acidic the oxygen level of the body decreases and this will reduce the rate of cellular metabolism. This can promote the growth of cancer cells. Alkaline environment promotes the growth of healthy cells and prevent the formation of cancer cells.

- Alkaline foods make your teeth and gums healthier. When the pH of the body becomes acidic the bacteria growth in the mouth increases and this leads to bad breath and various gum diseases. Acidity in the mouth promotes tooth decay. When you follow an alkaline diet your oral health will improve.

- The alkaline diet helps to reduce pain and inflammation of the joints. One of the minerals needed for neutralizing the acidic environment is magnesium. When your body becomes acidic the body will need more magnesium to neutralize it. Our body needs magnesium to support the joints and tissue functions. When the body uses the magnesium to neutralize acidity the joints and tissues will not get enough magnesium. The alkaline diet will make the environment alkaline and magnesium will be available to the joints which reduces the pain and inflammations.

- It has been found that the alkaline diet makes the cells to function more efficiently and the body will be able to produce new cells and repair the cells more efficiently. This will prevent premature aging.

Some Alkaline-Forming Foods

- Root vegetables- Root vegetables such as beets, carrots; radish, turnip and rutabaga are rich in minerals compared to many other vegetables available. You can use steamed root vegetables as part of your alkaline diet.

- Leafy greens- Leafy greens such as spinach, kale, turnip greens and Swiss chard are packed with vitamins, antioxidants, minerals and fiber. Spinach is a rich source of vitamin k and folate.

- Cruciferous Vegetables- Cruciferous vegetables such as cabbage, cauliflower, broccoli and Brussels sprouts are alkaline forming foods which are rich in fiber.

- Garlic- Garlic is an alkaline-forming food which improves overall health as they promote immune responses, cleanses the liver, promotes cardiovascular health and helps to maintain blood pressure.

- Lemons- This is the most powerful alkalizing food. It has antibacterial properties and can heal wounds. It helps the body to fight infections caused by bacteria and viruses. It promotes the detoxification of the liver.

- Cayenne peppers- This food contains enzymes which are necessary for proper endocrine function. They are a rich source of vitamin A they also fight off the free radicals formed in our body.

- Dry fruits – Dry fruits like dates, figs and apricots are rich in minerals like iron which is necessary for hemoglobin production. This will improve the oxygen carrying capacity of the blood.

- Nuts- Almonds, walnut and pecans contain useful fats which are necessary for the proper functioning of the body.

Top Alkaline Rich Food Recipes

Here are some recipes of alkaline-forming food preparations which will help you to balance your pH and improve your health quickly and without much effort. You can make adjustments in the recipes according to your taste and availability of items, but make sure that you are replacing the item with an alkaline –forming ingredient. The following are some of the best alkaline rich food recipes that you can try out to stay healthy, fit and to maintain a perfect pH balance level in your blood always.

This colorful, firm vegetable salad is not just pleasing for the eyes, but is also a very tasty and healthy salad. In fact, the Spanish bean salad can be custom made depending on the veggies that you like cucumber, avocado or tomatoes. It is not just the veggies that you can custom add, you can also think of adding the bean varieties that you like to make a tasty and delicious healthy salad.

Ingredients

- One can of pinto beans (rinsed properly and drained)

- One can of cannellini beans (rinsed and drained properly)

- One can of chick peas (rinsed and drained)

- 2 medium sized peeled carrots (diced into small cubes)

- 1 chopped red bell pepper

- 2 celery stalks, finely chopped

- ½ cup olive oil for tossing

- 2 green onions, finely chopped

- 2 tbsp lemon juice

- 1 or 2 cloves of finely chopped garlic

- ¼ cup cilantro, finely chopped

- ½ tbsp freshly ground cumin powder

- 1 tsp ground black pepper

- 1 tsp red chili powder

- Sea Salt and cayenne pepper for seasoning

Procedure

- Take a large bowl and add the beans, chopped and diced vegetables and green onions and toss them.

- Now in another small bowl, add olive oil, black pepper powder, cumin powder, chili powder, garlic, lemon juice and sea salt. Whisk all these ingredients together so that they mix well.

- Now pour the salad dressing over the beans and veggie mixture and combine it in such a way that the beans do not get mashed.

- Serve the Spanish bean salad over fresh greens and enjoy it for lunch or dinner.

Another healthy and tasty veggie salad that you can think of is the summer coleslaw. It is a crunchy and tasty salad that is rich in potassium, calcium, sodium and magnesium, which are the essential and vital alkaline minerals needed to maintain the pH balance.

Ingredients

- 3 medium sized carrots, de-skinned and julienne cut

- 2 cups of thinly sliced red cabbage

- 2 cups of finely sliced Naga cabbage

- 2 cups of bok choy that are sliced (use both white and green parts)

- 2 medium sized red bell peppers (finely sliced)

Dressing

- 2 tbsp extra virgin organic olive oil

- 1 tbsp lemon juice

- 2 tbsp Braggs liquid aminos

- 2 tsp ginger (grated)

- 1 tbsp toasted sesame oil

- 2 tsp raw sesame

- Sea salt and black pepper powder for seasoning

Procedure

- Take a nice large glass bowl ad put all the finely sliced veggies in the bowl and mix them gently. Make sure that you do not mix the veggies with a lot of force as they are very finely sliced.

- Whisk together all the dressing components in an other bowl.

- Pour the dressing over the mixed finely sliced veggies and toss it well so that the dressing is evenly coated on the veggie mixture.

- Serve immediately.

Special Raw Veggie Soup

If you would love to maintain the pH levels in your body at optimum levels, then you need to take in foods that are rich in alkali. All veggies have a high alkaline content and hence you need to consume them in a raw state or as a soup to enjoy its various health benefits.

Ingredients

- 2 cups of roughly chopped carrots

- 1 small avocado

- ½ cup frozen or fresh peas (make sure that the frozen peas are defrosted)

- juice of one small lime

- 1 tablespoon finely chopped shallot

- ½ inch piece ginger

- 2 cups of plain water

- ½ tsp sea salt

- Fresh finely chopped cilantro and hazelnut oil for garnish

Preparation

- Put all the veggies, juices, water and salt in a high speed blender.

- Run the blender on low speed for about one minute or so and slowly increase the speed levels of the blender.

- Keep it running on high for about 3 to 4 minutes or until all the veggies and juices are mixed through to make a smooth paste.

- Now pour the extract into warmed soup bowls and garnish it with fresh cilantro and a drizzle of hazelnut oil. Consume this soup raw to get a healthy punch of live enzymes, vitamins and minerals.

You can make a yummy cocktail or dessert by using Rhubarb, apples and beets. You will be able to easily make a thick, sweetened and intense flavored pudding using these three ingredients. It offers you the right sweet and sour taste that will linger on your tongue for long. Moreover, it is a very healthy and nutritious drink that is loaded with vitamins and minerals.

Ingredients

- 3 cups of chopped rhubarb

- Juice of 1 beet

- Juice of 2 apples

- ½ tsp vanilla essence

- 3 drops of liquid stevia

- 1/3 cup of chia seeds

- 1 tsp agave syrup

- 30 ml of filtered water

Procedure

- Add the freshly prepared apple juice along with the chopped rhubarb in a small casserole.

- Mix them well and then bake this mixture at 375 degrees for about 30 minutes or until the rhubarb becomes tender. Make sure that stir the mixture one or two times when it is getting prepared.

- Now once it is done, you need to allow it to cool for about 30 minutes until it is just a little warm.

- Add chia seeds, fresh beet juice and vanilla essence and mix it well. Allow it to react for about 10 minutes and no longer.

- Now take this mixture and put it in a blender. Blend the mixture on high speed until the chia seeds get completely smooth. You can add one or two tablespoons of filtered water if you want consistency.

- Add liquid stevia for sweetness and also agave syrup for the tartness.

- Scoop it out into dessert dishes and serve it either chilled or as it is.

- This special pudding will last for about three days under refrigeration.

- You can also prepare a special cocktail by blending rhubarb, beets and apple together in a blender and straining this mixture into a cocktail glass.

This salad contains many alkaline –forming ingredients such as kale, garlic, almonds, sunflower seeds, paprika, etc. You will see your cholesterol level drop after you take this salad regularly. This salad will improve your metabolic rate.

Ingredients

- large bunch of Kale

- 1 cup sunflower seeds (keep aside 1 teaspoon of seeds for garnishing)

- 1/3 cup raw almond nuts

- 1/8 tsp chipotle powder or according to the taste (Add more if you want to make it spicy)

- 1/2 tsp smoked paprika

- garlic cloves

- 1 1/4 cup water

- 1 1/2 tsp agave syrup (substitute with rice malt syrup if you want to avoid sugar)

- 1/2 tsp sea salt

Procedure

- Wash and pat dry the kale leaves.

- Remove the center membrane just up to where it thins out; tear the kale leaf into smaller pieces. Place the kale in a very large bowl.

- Put all the remaining ingredients into blender and blend until the mix becomes creamy and smooth.

- Pour half of this mixture over the kale leaves. Now toss the ingredients so that kale gets coated with the cream. Add remaining mixture and ensure that folds and curls of the leaves are coated.

- Allow this mix to stand for 10 minutes to tenderize the kale leaves.

- Plate the greens and sprinkle with sunflower seeds to garnish it.

Rainbow Salad

The name says it all. This salad is prepared with a wide array of colorful vegetables and hence the name. This salad is packed with enough dosage of goodness as well as offers the necessary alkalization that your body needs. It is loaded with Vitamins A, B and C along with essential nutrients and minerals.

Ingredients

- 1 yellow beet (grated and also cut in spiral shape)
- 2 carrots, ribboned using a peeler
- A small red onion, thinly sliced
- 6 yellow bell pepper slices
- 1 sliced avocado
- Pea shoots, sprouts
- Baby spinach leaves or small arugulas
- Chopped raw pistachios

Dressing

- 1 avocado
- One and half chopped red onion
- Juice of 2 meyer lemons

- 6 stems of fresh dill

- 6 basil leaves

- 1/3rd cup of extra virgin olive oil (cold pressed)

- 3 drops of stevia sweetener

- Sea salt to taste

Preparation

- In a salad bowl, place a handful of arugula or baby spinach leaves at the base. Now add the beets and other veggies and then ad the pea shoots and sprouts and finally top the salad with green pistachios.

- You need to take the dressing ingredients in a bowl and mix them well. Then, put this mixture in a high sped blender and process it until it gets creamy.

- Pour the required amount of the dressing on the prepared salad and toss it well.

- The sumptuous rainbow salad is ready to be served.

Using soaked sprouts and lentils in this recipe will provide a lot of nutrition and will help in waking up the living enzymes in your body. It will help in increasing body immunity as well as will aid in digestion.

Ingredients

- ½ cup pre-soaked, sprouted lentils

- 4 sun dried tomatoes that are finely diced and packed in olive oil

- 1 ½ cup of vegetable broth

- 1/3 rd cup of finely chopped or minced shallots or white onions

- 3 cloves of minced or finely chopped garlic

- 1 cup diced tomatoes

- 1 tsp fresh ginger (grated)

- 2 cups of finely chopped fresh spinach

- 2 cups of finely chopped baby kale

- 1 tbsp extra virgin coconut oil

- 50 ml of filtered water

- Extra virgin olive oil for drizzling

- Freshly ground pepper and Himalayan salt for seasoning

Preparation

- Cook the pre-soaked, sprouted lentils in the vegetable broth that you freshly prepared. You can also use organic vegetable broth cube to prepare the broth. Boil the lentils in the broth on high flame, then cover the broth solution with a lid and simmer it on low flame for about 20 minutes.

- Allow the water to get nearly absorbed and then turn off the heat.

- In a sauté pan, now add chopped onions and garlic and sauté them on medium heat till the onions become translucent.

- Now add the diced fresh tomatoes as well as the sun dried tomatoes along with 2 to 3 tablespoons of filtered water on high heat until the water bubbles.

- Now reduce the heat to low and simmer until the tomatoes melt.

- At this point, add the grated ginger and stir well for two minutes.

- Now add the freshly chopped baby spinach leaves along with 2 tablespoons of filtered water. Bring this mixture to a boil and then simmer on low flame until the green melts.

- Now add the cooked lentils and stir everything so that they mix properly.

- Serve this special healthy dish on a serving plate along with a small salad and eat it hot.

If you are looking to cleanse your system to stay healthy and free from digestion problems, then having this green raw veggie soup is a great idea. Drinking about 3 liters of water along with the raw green soup in a day will help you to easily remove all the toxins and unwanted wastes from your body. You can take this veggie soup ad water diet for three days on a stretch to get rid of all the toxins.

Ingredients

- 1 small zucchini, finely chopped

- 1 avocado

- 2 stalks of fresh celery, finely chopped

- 2 cups of spinach (raw)

- ½ cup of fresh cilantro

- ¼ cup of fresh parsley

- 1 minced clove of garlic

- 1 tbsp of finely chopped raw onion

- 2 green pepper slices

- ¼ cup of overnight soaked and rinsed raw almonds

- Fresh juice of one lime

- 1 ½ cups of pure water

- Sea salt to taste

Procedure

- Add all the ingredients other than the sea salt in a high speed blender and blend them together. Make sure that you add the required amounts of pure water to get the required consistency for the soup.

- Now transfer the raw veggie soup into a saucepan and warm the soup gently on low heat.

- Make sure that the soup is just warm and not hot.

- Add sea salt for seasoning as well as lime juice to flavor the soup.

- Serve it in a soup bowl in the warm state.

To maintain a healthy body, you need to take al least one green drink every day. One of the easiest green drinks that you can make is the green lemonade juice.

Ingredients

- 2 large kale leaves

- A small English cucumber

- 1 peeled lemon

- 1 apple

Preparation

- Add all the above ingredients in a blender and run it on slow speed first for about 30 seconds. Then run it on medium speed for about 20 seconds and then put it on high speed for about 2 minutes until the mixture becomes smooth.

- Add pure water to make it a bit light.

- Now strain the mixture through a strainer into a tall juice glass and consume immediately or after keeping it in a refrigerator for some time.

www.ingramcontent.com/pod-product-compliance
Lightning Source LLC
Chambersburg PA
CBHW061948280526
45787CB00004B/1775